Wiem BARBARIA

Hyaline membrane disease in term newborns

Wiem BARBARIA

Hyaline membrane disease in term newborns

Myth or reality?

ScienciaScripts

Imprint

Any brand names and product names mentioned in this book are subject to trademark, brand or patent protection and are trademarks or registered trademarks of their respective holders. The use of brand names, product names, common names, trade names, product descriptions etc. even without a particular marking in this work is in no way to be construed to mean that such names may be regarded as unrestricted in respect of trademark and brand protection legislation and could thus be used by anyone.

Cover image: www.ingimage.com

This book is a translation from the original published under ISBN 978-620-6-71247-3.

Publisher:
Sciencia Scripts
is a trademark of
Dodo Books Indian Ocean Ltd. and OmniScriptum S.R.L publishing group

120 High Road, East Finchley, London, N2 9ED, United Kingdom
Str. Armeneasca 28/1, office 1, Chisinau MD-2012, Republic of Moldova, Europe
Printed at: see last page
ISBN: 978-620-7-65473-4

HYALINE MEMBRANE DISEASE IN TERM NEWBORNS: MYTH OR REALITY?

DR WIEM BARBARIA

TABLE OF CONTENTS

INTRODUCTION

Hyaline membrane disease is a respiratory condition characterised by a qualitative or quantitative insufficiency of pulmonary surfactant [1]. This surface-active substance, secreted by type 2 pneumocytes, is essential for normal respiratory function.While surfactant deficiency is a well-known entity in premature newborns, it remains little-known or even denied in newborns whose gestational age is greater than or equal to 37 weeks' gestation. However, several studies and publications report the existence of respiratory pathology with clinical, radiological and even biological characteristics of MMH in term newborns. Thus, this entity is not so exceptional in the NNAT.Diagnosis is based on clinical and radiological criteria [2]. Intensive care management of full-term neonates presenting with respiratory distress syndrome must take into account the possibility of a diagnosis of MMH in order to avoid delayed diagnosis and therefore delayed management, which can sometimes be fatal. In fact, early administration of exogenous surfactant c a n improve the prognosis of these babies, who are usually born with severe respiratory distress. Certain circumstances may favour the onset of this disease in newborns at term. Male sex, mode of delivery and caesarean section before the onset of labour have been incriminated [3,4].

The objectives of our study were:

1- To determine the epidemiological, clinical and evolutionary profile of respiratory distress associated with hyaline membrane disease in full-term newborns.

2- Identify the factors predisposing to this pathology in order to establish a diagnosis. care and prevention strategy.

METHODS

1- Type of study

We conducted a retrospective descriptive study in the neonatology and neonatal intensive care unit of the main military training hospital in Tunis. This is a level 3 maternity unit.

2- Population study

We collated newborns who presented with respiratory distress whose retained aetiological diagnosis was MMH, admitted to our department over a 3-year period spanning between 1er January 2014 and 31 December 2016. Newborns admitted from the birth room of the gynaecology-obstetrics department of the main military training hospital in Tunis are called "In born". Out born" newborns are transferred to our department from another public or private health facility after prior telephone agreement.

2-1- Inclusion criteria

During the study period, we included all newborns whose gestational age was greater than or equal to 37 completed weeks of amenorrhoea, established by the theoretical calculation of the term from the first day of the last menstrual period or from the data of the early ultrasound examination performed before 12 weeks of amenorrhoea, whenever this examination was carried out.

Clinical of term à the birth by morphological criteria was used as a secondary criterion for assessing term.

2-2- Non-inclusion criteria

Our study did not include all newborns whose gestational age was strictly less than 37 weeks of amenorrhoea by theoretical calculation of the term or by estimation based on morphological criteria, or all newborns with a malformative pathology diagnosed ante- or post-natally.

3- Diagnostic criteria for hyaline membrane disease

3-1- Clinical criteria

The diagnosis of MMH was made whenever the newborn presented early-onset respiratory distress with signs of retraction from the first hour of life, with progressively worsening oxygen dependence associated or not with cyanosis. Blood cultures from the first 72 hours were negative.

3-2- Radiological criteria

The diagnosis of MMH was made on frontal chest X-rays.

if at least two of the following signs are present:
- Low pulmonary expansion
- A diffuse alveolar syndrome with a homogeneous reduction in the transparency of the lung parenchyma

- An air bronchogram

4- Data collection clinical

We consulted the medical records of newborns admitted to our department during the study period and completed a form containing the following information (Appendix 1):

- Data relating to the mother: age, parity and pathological history
- Data relating to the progress and monitoring of the pregnancy
- Data relating to childbirth
- Data relating to the newborn :
- Examination in the delivery room: Apgar (Appendix 2) and Silvermann score (Appendix 3)

- Care in the delivery room for patients in born
- Intensive care unit management
- Evolution and future

5- Definitions

5-1- Poverty

A paucipare is a woman who has given birth to two or three newborn babies. born with a gestational age greater than or equal to 28 SA.

5-2- Multiparity

A multiparous woman was considered to be any woman who had given birth to four or more babies with a gestational age greater than 28 weeks' gestation.

5-3- Premature rupture of the membranes

The diagnosis of RPM was evoked whenever the parturient reported a liquid vaginal discharge, the vaginal pH was alkaline after the discharge and the ultrasound showed a decrease in the amount of amniotic fluid compared with previous ultrasounds.

5-4- Fever

We defined maternal fever as any parturient whose rectal temperature was above 38.5°C during labour or 6 hours after delivery. In newborns, hyperthermia was defined as a rectal temperature above 38°C.

5-5- Macrosomia

Macrosomic newborns are those whose birth weight was strictly greater than 4000g.

5-6- Intrauterine growth retardation

Intrauterine growth retardation was defined as a birth weight below the 10ème percentile according to the Leroy and Lefort reference curves.

5-7- Excess intrauterine development

Excess intrauterine development was defined as a birth weight of

greater than the 97ème percentile according to the Leroy and Lefort reference curves.

5-8- Eutrophy

A newborn was eutrophic when its birth weight was between the 10ème and 97ème percentile.

5-9- Pulmonary arterial hypertension :

The diagnosis of PAH was made in respiratory unstable neonates with high oxygen requirements and a saturation difference of more than 15% between the supraductal and subductal levels. The diagnosis was confirmed by cardiac ultrasound whenever the systemic arterial pressure measured at the trunk of the pulmonary artery was greater than 50 mmHg.

5-10- Hemodynamic disorders :

The haemodynamic status of neonates was altered if the recolouring time was prolonged beyond 3 seconds, associated with tachycardia with or without oliguria.

5-11- Healthcare-associated infections :

We suspected healthcare-associated infection in newborns who had a change in complexion, haemodynamic problems beyond 48 hours after admission, abnormal haemograms with or without elevated C-reactive protein, or positive cultures from peripheral or central samples or prostheses.

6- Analysis statistics

The data were analysed using SPSS statistical software. version 17.0. Categorical variables were described in terms of numbers and percentages, and qualitative variables were described in terms of numbers and percentages. continuous quantitative variables by the mean ± standard deviation.

7- **Ethical considerations and conflicts of interest**

We have complied with all ethical considerations and are not reporting any conflict of interest.

RESULTS

Epidemiological, clinical and evolutionary profile of the disease of hyaline membranes in term newborns Results

1- Epidemiological study

1-1 Frequency :

The neonatology and neonatal intensive care unit of the HMPIT recorded 272 admissions of full-term neonates presenting with neonatal respiratory distress during the study period. MMH was diagnosed in 34 of these admissions, a frequency of 12.5%. The distribution of admissions is shown in table 1.

Table I: Breakdown of admissions during the study period

Year	Number of admissions	Number of NNAT*s	Number of NN** included
2014	1184	117	12
2015	1154	53	09
2016	1009	102	13

* NNAT: newborns at term, ** NN: newborns.

1-2- Data

1-2-1- Maternal age

The average age of the mothers was 33.18±4.6 years, with extremes between 27 and 43 years. The most common age group was between 27 and 34 (Figure 1).

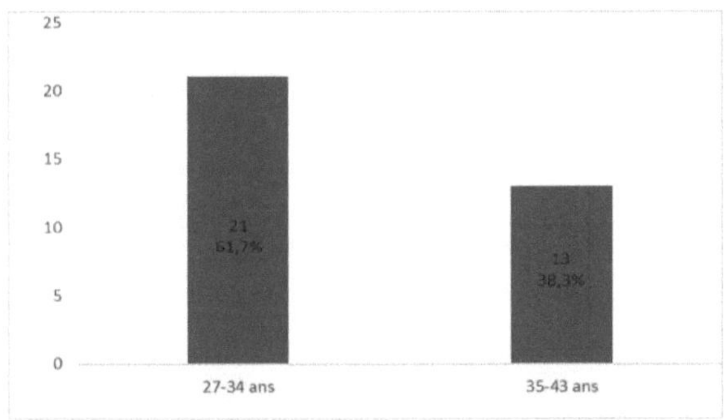

Figure 1: Breakdown of mothers by age group

1-2-2- Parity

The mean parity was 2.56±1.02 with extremes between 1 and 5. The majority of women were poor (Figure 2).

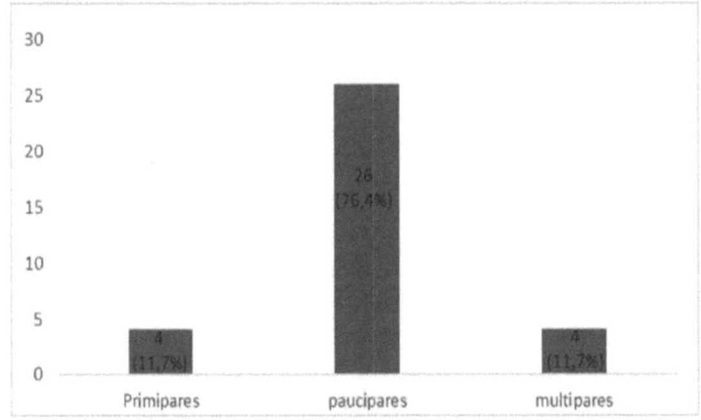

Figure 2: Distribution of mothers by parity

1-2-3- Maternal pathology

The majority of the women had no particular medical history. Four had hypothyroidism and two had type 1 diabetes. Only one of the following conditions was noted: asthma, hepatitis B, arterial hypertension and breast nodule (Table 2).

Table II: Breakdown of maternal pathologies

Pathology	No pathologies	Hypo-thyroid disease	Diabetes type 1	asthma	Hepatitis B	HTA*	Breast nodule
n	24	4	2	1	1	1	1
%	70,7%	11,8%	5,8%	2,9%	2,9%	2,9%	2,9%

*hypertension: high blood pressure

1-2-4- Pregnancy progress and monitoring

- All the pregnancies were spontaneous, monochorionic and well monitored.

- All women were screened for gestational diabetes. It was present in 7 women.

- Elevated blood pressure during pregnancy was found in only 3 women.

- Dexamethasone-based antenatal corticosteroid therapy was administered to three women, only one of whom received two full courses and two of whom received a single course.

- Amniotic fluid was clear in 32 women. One woman had stained fluid and one woman had meconium fluid.

- Premature rupture of the membranes was found in three women.
- Fetal heart rate recording was normal in all pregnancies except in one case where the trace showed fetal tachycardia.

- Maternal fever of 38.8°C was present in only one woman.

1-3- Neonatal data

1-3-1- Place of delivery

The majority of newborns included in our study were "out born" with a frequency of 58.9%. The distribution of newborns according to place of delivery is shown in Figure 3.

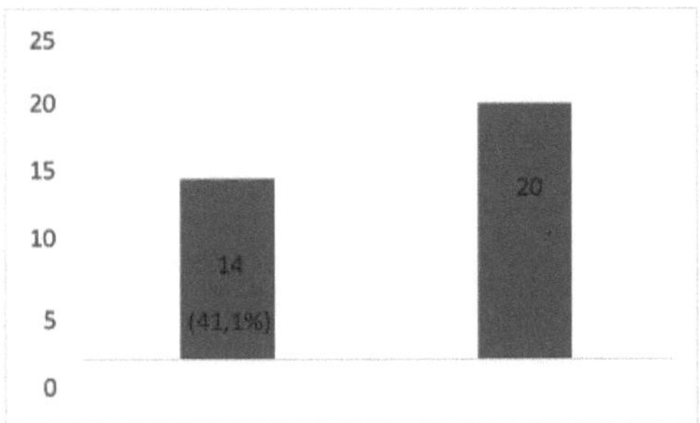

Figure 3 : Distribution of newborns by place of delivery

1-3-2- Breakdown by gender

We noted a male predominance of NNATs admitted to our department for neonatal respiratory distress related to MMH during the study period, with a sex ratio of 1.6 (Figure 4).

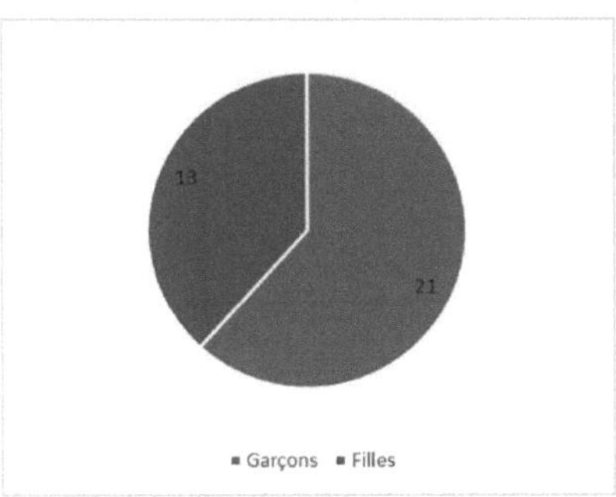

Figure 4: Breakdown of newborn babies by sex

This male predominance was found for both in-born and out-born babies (Figure 5).

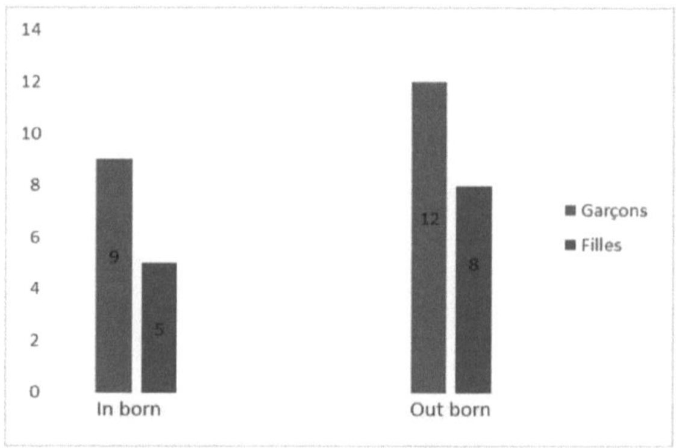

Figure 5 : Gender distribution by place of birth

1-3-3- Gestational age at birth

The mean gestational age at birth was 38.12±0.96 SA with extremes between 37 and 41 SA. The distribution of births by gestational age is shown in the table below. figure 6.

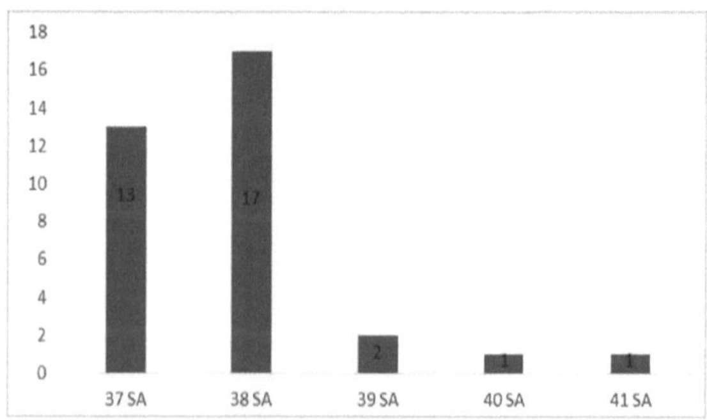

Figure 6 : Distribution of births by gestational age

1-3-4- Mode of delivery

The majority of newborns were delivered by the vaginal route. Cold caesarean section was planned in 28 women. Emergency caesarean section was indicated in 3 women for the following reasons: spontaneous onset of labour in a scarred uterus, chorioamniotitis and severe pre-eclampsia. Only three women had a non-instrumental vaginal delivery.

2- Study clinical

2-1- Apgar

All the newborns had adapted well to life outside the womb. The mean Apgar at 5 minutes was 9.51±0.75 with extremes between 7 and 10.

2-2- Birth weight

The mean birth weight was 3306±520 g with extremes between 2170 and 4600 g. Macrosomia was present in three newborns. Only two babies had a birth weight of less than 2500 g. The majority of newborns were eutrophic. Five had intrauterine growth retardation and two had excess intrauterine development. The distribution of birth weights according to gestational age is shown in Figure 7.

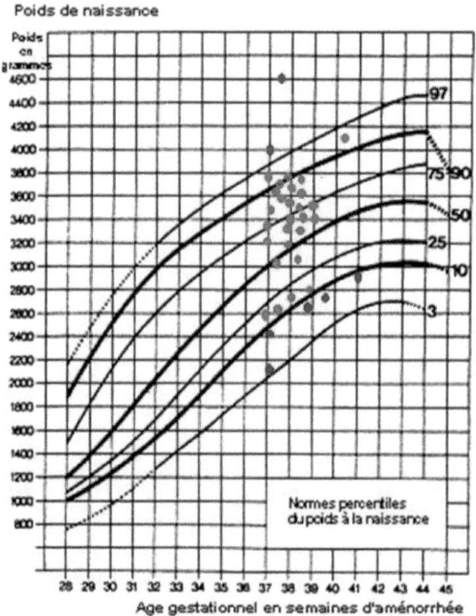

Figure 7: Distribution of birth weights by gestational age.

2-3- Age of newborns at on admission

The mean age of neonates on admission was 12.05±14.25 hours [1- 48]. The "out born" were aged 19.15±14.43 hours [2-48]. The mean age of "in born" was 1.57±1.09 [1-4].

2-4- Clinical manifestations

- Respiratory distress was immediate in all neonates.
- Cyanosis was present in 12 newborns (35.2%).
- The mean respiratory rate was 70.41±15.93 cpm [40-120].
- The mean Silvermann score on admission was 4.46±1.57 [2-6].
- The Silvermann score was greater than 4 in 22 newborns (64.7%).

- The mean transcutaneous oxygen saturation on admission measured by pulse oximeter was 87.08±12.48% [60-100%].

- Haemodynamic disorders with a recolouring time of more than 3 seconds were present in 13 neonates (38.2%).

- Neurological manifestations such as hypotonia were present in 4 newborns (11.7%).

- Four newborns had problems with temperature regulation, including 3 with hyperthermia.

-

2-5- Imaging

All neonates had a full-face chest X-ray taken in the intensive care unit at the patient's bedside. The average time taken to obtain chest X-rays was 10.85±12.43 hours, with extremes of between 1 and 43 hours. The majority of radiographs showed an alveolar syndrome. Intra-thoracic gas effusion was present in six cases (Figure 8).

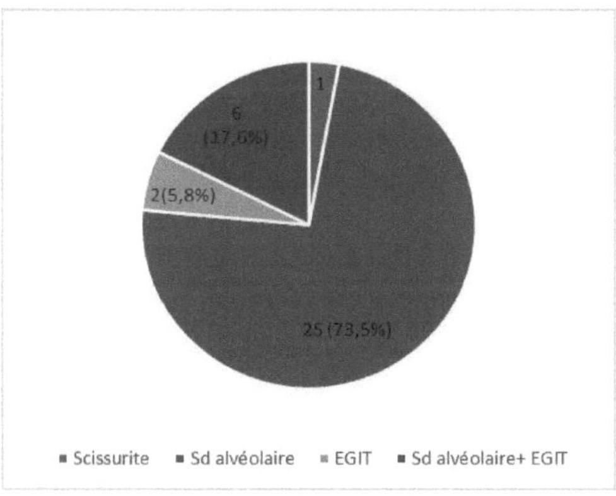

Figure 8: Radiographic findings in neonates on admission.

2-6- Blood gasometry

Blood gases were measured in all neonates. The average time taken to perform blood gas measurements was 14.59±15.08 hours, with extremes of between 0.5 and 50 hours.The mean pH on admission was 7.32±0.10 [7.14-7.52]. The average partial pressure of carbon dioxide on admission was 34.04±10.07 mmHg [19-62].

3- Available at

3-1- Treatment symptomatic

All neonates had received initial or first hour oxygen therapy using Hood's enclosure. The indications were polypnoea in 8 neonates, signs of struggle in 24 and combination of polypnoea with signs of struggle in two neonates. The mean duration of Hood oxygen therapy was 11.94±12.53 hours [0.5-47].Non-invasive nasal ventilation was indicated in 19 neonates. The mean age of NIV use was 13.5±21.98 hours [0.5-96]. The mean duration of NIV was 12.44±25.47 hours [1-114]. The indications for NIV were persistent signs of struggle or polypnoea in 14 newborns. and hypoxia for 5 neonates.

All neonates received mechanical ventilation. The indication was at a mean age of 16.88±14.46 hours [2-54].

The most frequent indication for mechanical ventilation was hypoxia with desaturation in 55.9% of cases. High oxygen requirements in excess of 40% were noted in 20.6% of neonates. Persistent signs of struggle were noted in 17.7% of neonates and EGIT in 5.8%. High-frequency oscillatory ventilation was indicated in 26.5% of cases at a mean age of 49.77±18.84 hours [24-75]. The indication was refractory hypoxaemia in all 25 cases. The mean duration was 47.66±44.37 hours [9-144].

3-2- Treatment

All neonates were treated with exogenous surfactant by instillation through the intubation tube. Treatment was administered at a mean age of 21.85±17.39 hours [3-76]. Only two neonates required a second instillation due to an increase in oxygen requirements above 40% twelve hours after the first instillation.

4- Complications :

4-1- Intra- thoracic gas effusions

The occurrence of EGIT complicated the management of 32.3% of newborns, 16% of which were pneumothorax requiring thoracic drainage. Pneumomediastinum occurred in 16.3%. EGIT was associated with non-invasive nasal ventilation in 3 neonates, with conventional mechanical ventilation in 4 neonates and with Hood oxygen therapy in 4 neonates.

4-2- Pulmonary arterial hypertension

Pulmonary arterial hypertension was found in 58% of cases. The use of inhaled nitric oxide was indicated for all cases of PAH at a mean age of 52.67±23.76 hours [52-90].

4-3- Disorders haemodynamics

Haemodynamic disorders with recourse to vasoactive drugs were noted in 70% of cases.

4-4- Infection associated with care

Broad-spectrum antibiotic therapy was indicated in 30% of newborns for suspected healthcare-associated infection. Bacteriological confirmation was obtained in 11.7% of cases.

5- Evolution

- The mean length of hospital stay was 10.17±7.6 days [1-34].
- In 64.7% of newborns, discharge was without sequelae.
- Convulsions and hypotonia were noted in 23.5% of cases.
- Four newborns died of pulmonary hypertension in 3 cases and DIC in one case, related to a healthcare-associated infection.

MMH in term newborns is a real entity. It has specific clinical, therapeutic and developmental features. The prognosis is usually good if the condition is managed early and the ventilatory strategy is adapted. In our study, the incidence of the disease was 12.5%. The majority of newborns included in our study were "out born". The sex ratio was 1.6. The mean gestational age was 38.12±0.96 SA. Gestational diabetes was present in 20.5% of cases. Insulin-dependent diabetes prior to pregnancy was present in 5.8% of women. The most frequent mode of delivery was a scheduled cold caesarean section outside labour in 82% of cases. The average age of newborns on admission was 12.05±14.25 hours. The "out born" were 19.15±14.43 hours old. The mean age of the inborns was 1.57±1.09 hours. Respiratory distress was immediate in all newborns, with cyanosis in 35.2% of cases. Chest X-rays showed an alveolar syndrome in 91.1% of cases. EGIT was present in 17.6% of cases. All neonates underwent mechanical ventilation at a mean age of 16.88±14.46 hours, with treatment with exogenous surfactant at a mean age of 21.85±17.39 hours. The outcome was favourable in 88.2% of cases, with 64% of neonates discharged without sequelae.Few studies have investigated MMH in the term newborn. This may be explained by the difficulty of eliminating other pathologies with the same clinico-radiological characteristics as MMH. Infectious alveolitis or transient respiratory distress are more easily evoked. The limitations of our work were the retrospective nature of the study, with a lack of precision in certain medical record data. The heterogeneity of the study population and the inclusion of "out born" newborns led to a selection bias, resulting in an overestimate of the frequency of this condition in our department. Finally, the non-availability of fetal lung maturation tests in utero in our study, which are not in common practice in gynaecology departments in general.

1- Pathophysiology of hyaline membrane disease

The term hyaline membrane disease refers to the histological aspect of the most common pulmonary pathology in premature newborns. It is linked to a qualitative or quantitative insufficiency of pulmonary surfactant. Surfactant deficiency and the immature lung structure with reduced alveolisation in the premature newborn produce alveolar instability, haemorrhagic oedema, inflammation with necrosis of the alveoli leading to the formation of characteristic eosinophilic hyaline deposits (hyaline membranes) which invade the terminal bronchi and alveolar ducts [1]. The membranes may reabsorb and the disease is cured by day 4ème or 5ème . However, MMH or its respiratory complications can be fatal in 2 to 3 days as a result of anoxia and acidosis. Surfactant is secreted by type 2 pneumocytes. The first lamellar inclusions (an intracellular form of surfactant secretion by type 2 pneumocytes) appear in humans between 20 and 24 days' gestation, but it is not until around 34-36 days' gestation that they actually become functional, forming a monolayer film that lines the surface of the pulmonary alveoli [6].

This is a multimolecular complex consisting essentially of phospholipids, neutral lipids and specific apoproteins. Phospholipids are the biochemical support for surfactant capacity. The function of proteins is to direct phospholipids to the alveolar interface in an effective functional form, thanks to protein-phospholipid and protein-protein molecular interactions [6].Surfactant maturation is subject to complex regulation via certain hormones, particularly glucocorticoids, and interactions with mesenchymal cells [6]. The main functions of surfactant are to reduce interface tension, stabilise alveoli of unequal size, prevent collapse of the alveoli and bronchioles at the end of exhalation, reduce the work of breathing, increase lung compliance and therefore create a functional residual capacity [6]. In the premature newborn who has not completed the maturation process of the various pulmonary constituents, none of these functions is actually present.

2- Pathophysiology of hyaline membrane disease in term newborns

Surfactant synthesis and secretion is regulated by a number of factors, mainly hormonal. Some of these factors slow down surfactant secretion, while others promote its synthesis and secretion.

2-1- Insulin

Gestational diabetes induces foetal hyperglycaemia, a source of foetal hyperinsulinism. It has been reported that insulin slows the maturation and secretion of pulmonary surfactant by two mechanisms: a defect in the synthesis of dipalmytoyl-phosphatidylcholine due to altered glycogen metabolism secondary to hyperinsulinism, and a direct antagonistic effect of insulin on glucocorticoids [7]. Clinical data assessing the impact of maternal diabetes on neonatal respiratory pathology are contradictory. The delay in lung maturation seems to be linked above all to maternal glycaemic control.

Correct glycaemic control reduces the risk of MMH in the newborn. According to a French study conducted at the Robert-Debré hospital, maternal diabetes treated with insulin, combined with other perinatal factors, was associated with a significantly greater risk of severe respiratory distress [8]. In multivariate analysis, newborns of diabetic mothers treated with insulin had an increased risk of severe respiratory distress in relation to MMH, independently of gestational age and mode of delivery (Odds ratio = 1.44 [1.00-2.08]) [8].

A Spanish study looked at the outcome of macrosomic newborns from pregnancies complicated or uncomplicated by gestational diabetes. It was shown that newborns whose mothers were treated with insulin were at greater risk of developing respiratory distress and, in particular, MMH [9].

According to the report of the French national perinatal survey published in 2010 [10], gestational diabetes was present in 7.2% of women, irrespective of the mode of management. Insulin-dependent diabetes was present in 1.7% of women. In Canada, the prevalence of gestational diabetes recorded in 2010 was 5.6% [11].

In our study, gestational diabetes was present in 20.5% of cases. Insulin-dependent diabetes prior to pregnancy was present in 5.8% of women. The high values found in our study compared with the data in the literature are due to the fact that our work was carried out in a level 3 maternity unit, where most of the management concerns pathological and high-risk pregnancies. In addition, most of the newborns included in our study were "outborns" who accumulate certain pregnancy-related morbidity factors, in particular diabetes. Thus, in addition to the small size of our sample, the newborns in our study appear to be pre-selected, which explains the high rate of gestational diabetes.

2-2- Caesarean section outside labour

The neonatal respiratory morbidity associated with cold caesarean delivery is currently a matter of certainty. Several studies have shown an increase in the incidence of MMH in cases of caesarean delivery, and in particular caesarean delivery scheduled outside labour [12-19]. Compression of the foetal rib cage during passage through the birth canal is responsible for the expulsion of a third of the pulmonary fluid through the mouth [20]. This phase is absent during vaginal delivery, which results in an increase in residual lung volume and a decrease in surfactant secretion towards the alveolar surface. Furthermore, surfactant maturation and secretion are triggered by labour and promoted by β-adrenergic agents and prostaglandins released in response to the stress experienced by the foetus during labour [21]. Some authors have shown that respiratory morbidity is greater in cases of repeated cold caesarean sections. This risk increases proportionally with the number of caesarean sections before the start of labour. The pathophysiological mechanisms are not clearly elucidated [22,23]. The degree of lung maturation is assessed by measuring the lecithin/sphingomyelin (L/S) ratio in the amniotic fluid and by the FLM test (fetal lung maturity test). In the case of MMH, the (L/S) ratio is <2 and the FLM is <50.mg/g [24,25]. In a study published by Ayachi et al, MMH was diagnosed in 97 newborns with a mean gestational age of 37 weeks + 4 days. The FLM test performed in 40 newborns was < 50 mg/g, indicating pulmonary immaturity [26]. As a result, several studies currently recommend a gestational age greater than or equal to 39 days' gestation for fetal extraction by elective caesarean section [27-29]. In our study, 91.3% of newborns were delivered by cold caesarean section outside labour at a mean gestational age of 38.12±0.96 SA. The choice of route of extraction depends on a number of factors relating to the habits of the obstetric team, who may favour the upper route, especially if there is a history of caesarean delivery, in order to avoid the risks associated with vaginal delivery, or sometimes to the wishes of the parturient who "prefers" to give birth by caesarean section. These practices are mainly observed in the private health sector. Thus, the high rate of elective caesarean sections observed in our study is due to a recruitment bias. In fact, our work mainly involved out-born women.

2-3- Male

It is well established in several species that lung maturation, as measured by surfactant synthesis and secretion, is delayed in the male foetus compared with the female foetus [30,31]. In fact, the presence of androgens delays pulmonary surfactant production [32].

The male predominance of respiratory distress in general and MMH in particular, regardless of gestational age, has been reported by several authors [26,33]. The results of our study are consistent with the literature. The sex ratio for MMH was 1.6.

2-4- the thyrotropic hormone

Experimental studies have shown that thyroid hormones accelerate foetal lung maturation [34]: foetal thyroidectomy leads to a delay in lung maturation, whereas the administration of thyroid hormones accelerates it. Triiodothyronine stimulates surfactant synthesis, sensitises sodium transfer mechanisms, decreases fluid production, and reduces the risk of lung death. This improves cardiac output and increases foetal respiratory movements. The exact mechanism of action of TRH on maturation is unclear. A synergy of action with corticoids is likely [34].

3- Data from literature

Respiratory distress in the newborn is a frequent reason for admission to the neonatal intensive care unit. There are many aetiologies for respiratory distress in the newborn, depending on the context of delivery. MMH is a diagnosis that should usually be considered in premature newborns, with its incidence inversely proportional to gestational age. Beyond 37 weeks' gestation, this condition is far from exceptional. In the literature, few studies have demonstrated the existence of this condition in NNATs. In a French study, Ayachi et al [26] collated 97 newborns admitted for MMH over a 5-year period. The diagnosis was based on clinical, radiological and biological criteria. The authors concluded that this entity does exist in NNATs, since fetal lung maturation was not correlated with gestational age. In this study, some fetuses were not mature at 37-38 weeks' gestation. MMH was diagnosed mainly in cases of fetal extraction before the onset of labour and in cases of induction at around 37 weeks' gestation. Gouyon et al [35] studied the aetiologies of neonatal respiratory distress in a retrospective study of 14813 neonates with a gestational age between 37 and 38 SA and 50187 neonates born between 39 and 41 SA. The main causes of mechanical ventilation were transient respiratory distress, MMH and meconium inhalation, with incidences of 0.72 ‰ [95% CI: 0.53 ‰ - 0.96 ‰], 0.38 ‰ [95% CI: 0.25 ‰- 0.57 ‰] and 0.61 ‰ [95% CI: 0.44 ‰,-0.84 ‰], respectively. Progression in gestational age from 37 to 41 SA was associated with a significant decrease in the incidence of MMH and transient tachypnoea.MMH treated by mechanical ventilation or positive expiratory pressure concerned 3.5% of children aged 35-36 ADT, 0.49% of children aged 37-38 ADT and 0.08% of children aged 39-41 ADT [35]. Liu et al [36] have shown that HMM is not a rare disease in term neonates and is associated with higher mortality. Its clinical features differ from those of

MMH in preterm infants because of thoracic rigidity, and its onset was more likely to be complicated by multivisceral failure and PAH. Most patients required prolonged mechanical ventilation. In Tunisia, few authors have studied respiratory distress in NNAT. Among the aetiologies of respiratory distress, MMH was not mentioned as a separate entity in NNATs. In 2007, Bouziri et al [37] studied acute respiratory distress syndrome in term and near term neonates. The clinico-radiological definition of this syndrome is similar to that of MMH. In our series, 34 term neonates were admitted to intensive care for respiratory distress related to MMH over a period of 3 years. The incidence was 12.5%. This frequency seems high because of the small size of the sample and because our study was conducted in an intensive care unit that treats "outborns", hence the pre-selection of newborns.

4- Inherited surfactant disorders lung

MMH reflects a qualitative or quantitative functional deficiency in pulmonary surfactant. Inherited disorders of pulmonary surfactant metabolism constitute a heterogeneous and significant group of respiratory disorders. Thus, MMH in full-term newborns may be linked either to pulmonary 'immaturity' or to a functional deficiency in surfactant proteins. Mutations in surfactant protein genes lead to an abnormality in surfactant production, which is responsible for a toxic accumulation in type II pneumocytes. The administration of exogenous surfactant proves ineffective in the latter case, and the disease progresses to refractory hypoxaemia [5]. The identification of mutations in the genes encoding surfactant proteins has made it possible to explain the phenotypic variability of hereditary surfactant protein deficiency from birth to adulthood. Mutations in the SFTPB, SFTPC and ABCA3 genes encoding the SP-B, SP-C and ATP-binding cassette proteins respectively are the mutations responsible for MMH in newborns

[5]. Inherited SP-B deficiency was the first genetic cause of DRNN reported in the literature. The classic presentation is early respiratory distress (before the 12th hour of life) in term infants, with little or no response to treatment with exogenous surfactant and conventional ventilation [38,39]. More than 30 mutations in the SFTPB gene have been identified in patients with congenital SP-B deficiency.In humans, a mutation in SP-C was initially associated with neonatal respiratory disease very similar to that observed in SP-B deficiency [40]. More recently, several SP-C mutations have been shown to be responsible for chronic respiratory disease at different ages. The phenotype associated with SFTPC mutations is highly variable. Neonatal forms that can lead to death in the first few years of life, as well as late adult forms, have been observed. This variability in the age of onset of lung damage could be explained by the occurrence of environmental stresses, such as viral infection with the respiratory syncitial virus [41], or the association with mutations coding for other proteins involved in the synthesis of mature SP-C, such as SP-B or ABCA3 [42]. Thus, neonatal respiratory distress with the clinico-radiological features of MMH resistant to conventional treatment, whether or not associated with a family history, should raise the possibility of an inherited surfactant disorder. Unfortunately, in our country, the lack of resources for studying these genes makes it difficult to identify this pathology. As a result, some deaths are attributed to PAH without being able to study its aetiology.

5- Notion of surfactant deactivation syndrome

Secondary surfactant deficiency occurs in patients who initially have normal surfactant synthesis. Under the effect of various factors: infection, hypoxia, barovolotrauma from artificial ventilation, inhibiting factors reaching the alveolus, synthesis is reduced and the quality of the surfactant may be impaired with a reduction in the capacity to exchange respiratory gases [43].

In the study by Wax et al, a neonate aged 38 + 5 days developed MMH despite pulmonary maturation tests being performed on amniotic fluid prior to extraction by caesarean section [28]. This finding would seem to suggest an abnormality in surfactant acquisition after delivery. Some authors have proposed a test to detect surfactant dysfunction in the either by secondary deficiency or inactivation. The "Click test" involves taking a 0.2 ml tracheal sample and mixing it with 95% ethanol. The mixture forms bubbles and is examined under a microscope. If the bubbles increase and then decrease in size, the test is positive (active surfactant). If no bubbles are observed, the test is negative (surfactant inactive). The positive predictive value was 100% and the negative predictive value was 93% [44].

Other authors have proposed the "Gastric Shake Test", which involves taking 0.5 ml of gastric fluid within 20 minutes of birth, mixing it with an equal volume of saline solution for 15 seconds and 1 ml of 95% ethanol. The mixture is then shaken for 15 seconds. After standing for 15 min, the air-liquid interface was examined under a microscope. If no bubbles are present, the test is negative (very little surfactant is present). If bubbles are present directly on the fluid surface, then the test is positive (adequate amount of surfactant). Sensitivity was 100% and specificity 92% [45].

These tests are simple, rapid and inexpensive. They allow early diagnosis and faster recourse to surfactant treatment. In Tunisia, these tests are not available and are not commonly used, which makes MMH an underestimated entity. In our study, two neonates benefited from a second instillation of surfactant due to an increase in oxygen requirements above 40% twelve hours after the first instillation. This could be related either to a secondary deactivation of surfactant or, on the contrary, to an overestimation of the diagnosis of MMH and a rush to the initial administration of this product.

6- Prevention of hyaline membrane disease : Antenatal corticosteroid therapy

Glucocorticoids have a modulating effect on lung maturation. At the end of gestation, glucocorticoids increase the rate of phosphatidylcholine biosynthesis and therefore the quantity of phosphatidylcholine in the lung, as well as the activity of choline phosphate cytidyltransferase, a key enzyme in surfactant metabolism. Their effect on the biosynthesis and transcriptional activation of surfactant-specific protein genes is significant (SP-B and SP-C). The production of surfactant by pneumocytes II is thus facilitated [46,47]. Dexamethasone and betamethasone, which easily pass the placental barrier in active form and are weakly inactivated by 11ß-hydroxysteroid dehydrogenase, are indicated for the prevention of HMM. They improve the biomechanical characteristics of the animal lung (pressure/volume) and the surface-active properties of surfactant. They promote the incorporation of labelled precursors into the essential components of surfactant, in particular DPPC and phosphatidylglycerol. Above all, they induce an increase in the activity of numerous enzymes, in particular that of cytidylphosphocholine transferase CPCT, a key enzyme in phospholipid metabolism [46].

Several studies have demonstrated the efficacy of betamethasone in reducing the incidence of MMH in newborns under 34 weeks' gestation [48,49]. The incidence of MMH in newborns over 34 weeks' gestation is very low and, consequently, the difference between the treatment and control groups was not significant in the study by Bourbon et al: 2.5% versus 4.1% [50]. The benefit of antenatal corticosteroid therapy has been demonstrated with regard to the occurrence of MMH. Its incidence is significantly reduced by antenatal corticosteroid therapy. If this pathology occurs despite this prevention, it is less severe and the efficacy of exogenous surfactants is enhanced.According to some authors, corticosteroid therapy in the case of elective caesarean section reduces respiratory morbidity, mainly MMH, and avoids a stay in intensive care [51-53]. In a controlled English study, the incidence of neonatal respiratory distress was 18.7/1000 in a group of 373 term infants born by iterative caesarean section who received neonatal corticosteroid therapy, compared with 47.1/1000 in the control group (p=0.02). This supports the use of corticosteroid therapy whenever a delivery has to be induced, whatever the term, in order to reduce the incidence of respiratory distress in general and MMH in particular [54].

Saccone et al [55] published a meta-analysis of six randomised controlled trials evaluating the efficacy of antenatal corticosteroid therapy at 34 weeks' gestation in parturients whose delivery was planned by elective caesarean section. The The authors concluded that corticosteroids administered before a planned caesarean section at 37 weeks' gestation are effective in reducing respiratory distress syndrome. Corticosteroids should therefore be indicated whenever a caesarean section outside labour is possible at 37-38. At 39 weeks' gestation, the beneficial effects of corticosteroids are not certain.

In our study, antenatal corticosteroid therapy was only administered to three women, only one of whom received two full courses and two of whom received a single course at 34 weeks' gestation. This observation is a sad reality. There is no doubt about the benefit of antenatal corticosteroid therapy at 34 weeks' gestation. Obstetricians should systematically indicate courses of corticosteroids in all high-risk situations.

7- Management of hyaline membrane disease :

The diagnosis of MMH in newborns with a gestational age of more than 37 weeks presents a number of clinical and radiological particularities. In contrast to the premature newborn, the thoracic parietal osteocartilaginous structure is more rigid and the musculature is more developed in the term newborn. Thus, the signs of retraction assessed by the Silvermann index are less marked in the term neonate and only the expiratory whine, indicative of compliance problems, is almost constant and should lead to the diagnosis being made [56].

The Silvermann score, designed to assess the severity of respiratory distress syndrome in premature babies, is poorly adapted to term newborns in these circumstances. As a result, the use of this score in clinical practice leads to an underestimation of the severity of respiratory distress syndromes in NNATs and encourages delays in treatment. Transient respiratory distress is more easily diagnosed in NNATs.Radiologically, there is a moderate reduction in the transparency of the lung parenchyma due to the more efficient ventilatory efforts made by these children compared with premature infants. The classic image of microgranules with aerated bronchogram and alveolar syndrome is not always found [56].

These two phenomena are at the root of a delay in treatment, which must be avoided. This is based on oxygen therapy using mechanical ventilation with positive expiratory pressure and intra-tracheal instillation of exogenous surfactant [57].

In the study by Ayachi et al [26], the average time to care was 5 hours and the average time to admission to the intensive care unit was 10 hours. Goraya et al [58] reported in 2001 a case of MMH in a full-term newborn whose failure to recognise the diagnosis probably contributed to the newborn's death. The diagnosis was only made at autopsy.Curative treatment of MMH due to pulmonary immaturity must be given sufficiently early to ensure maximum efficacy of the product administered [59,60]. In a systematic review of the literature, the authors concluded that early administration of surfactant to neonates intubated before the third hour of life considerably enhances the surfactant effect and reduces the risk of complications and mortality [61].

It has also been shown that repeat administration of exogenous surfactant six to twelve hours after the first instillation may improve prognosis compared with single doses [62].

In our study, admission to the intensive care unit took place at a mean age of 12.05±14.25 hours. The mean admission time for out-born babies was 19.15±14.43 hours, and for in-born babies 1.57±1.09 hours.Neonates were mechanically ventilated at a mean age of 16.88±14.46 hours. Surfactant instillation was performed at a mean age of 21.85±17.39 hours. The delay in management in our series mainly concerned "outborns". This may be due to the fact that some maternity units do not have neonatology services and would have to transfer symptomatic newborns to another facility, which itself may not be able to provide intensive care management. Furthermore, once the agreement to transfer to our department has been given, the transport times and procedures cannot be controlled. This delay in care therefore represents a bias and does not allow us to extrapolate our results.

8- Complications

The management of neonates in respiratory distress in the intensive care unit carries a risk of complications inherent either in the pathology itself or in the therapies used. Intra thoracic gas effusions (pneumothorax and pneumomediastinum) and pulmonary arterial hypertension are the main complications of MMH whatever the term [63]. Some studies have shown a reduction in the incidence of respiratory and even neurological complications of MMH with the instillation of exogenous surfactant. According to a European study, early treatment with exogenous surfactant reduced the risk of pneumothorax (RR 0.68; 95% CI: 0.47 - 0.9) [64]. Hentschel et al [65] also showed a significant reduction in the risk of pneumothorax with early administration of surfactant (RR 0.69; 95% CI: 0.57-0.83).

In our study, the occurrence of EGIT complicated the management of 32.3% of neonates, 16% of whom had pneumothorax requiring thoracic drainage. Pneumomediastinum occurred in 16.3% of cases. In the study by Ayachi et al [26], pneumothorax was observed in 35% of cases. The aetiology of EGIT in the respiratory pathology of NNAT is multifactorial.EGIT was associated with non-invasive nasal ventilation in 3 neonates, with conventional mechanical ventilation in 4 neonates and with Hood oxygen therapy in 4 neonates.In addition, the surfactant deficiency observed in MMH induces hyperreactivity of the pulmonary arteries by alteration of the gas exchange mechanisms and thus predisposes these newborns to pulmonary hypertension [66].In an Egyptian study, PAH was a complication of HMM in 16.6% of cases were born by caesarean section [67].

In our study, PAH was found in 58% of cases. The use of nitric oxide was indicated in all cases of PAH at a mean age of 52.67±23.76 hours. Delayed management of MMH is a source of sometimes very serious complications. In our study, the delay in management mainly concerned"out born". EGIT and PAH were the main complications. This is in line with the data in the literature.

9- Mortality

The proportional neonatal mortality rate due to MMH reported in the literature is very heterogeneous. It was 15% in Sudan [68], 9.3% in India [69], 5.44% in China [70] and 1.16% in Italy [71]. This heterogeneity and wide variation in values can be explained by the development of hospital infrastructures and the immediate availability of resuscitation resources in developed countries such as Italy. The management of MMH in developing countries is not easy. The non-availability of ventilation machines and expensive exogenous surfactant are the main limiting factors, especially when it comes to neonates with several poor prognostic factors. In developing countries such as Tunisia, not all maternity units where babies are delivered at all stages have neonatal resuscitation services. In our study, the mortality rate for term newborns admitted to our department was 11.7%. This figure can be explained by the delay in diagnosis and management on the one hand, and by the potential seriousness of this disease on the other, especially when several risk factors are associated. Furthermore, this figure is overestimated due to the small size of the sample studied. Secondly, our maternity unit is a level 3 maternity unit which deals with serious pregnancy-related pathologies and high-risk pregnancies. Finally, the management of "outborns" in our department tends to increase mortality, since these newborns are pre-selected as potentially serious, hence the indication for transfer.

Hyaline membrane disease is a respiratory condition caused by a functional deficiency of pulmonary surfactant [1]. This substance, which essentially has surface-active properties, is essential for normal lung function. This pathology is well known in premature newborns, but is still poorly understood or even denied in term newborns. The diagnosis of MMH in a newborn whose gestational age is greater than 37 days' gestation should be made on the basis of anamnestic, clinical, radiological and sometimes biological criteria [2].Certain factors have been incriminated in the occurrence of this disease, principally male sex and delivery by cold caesarean section outside labour [3,4].

The objectives of our study were:

1- To determine the epidemiological, clinical and evolutionary profile of respiratory distress associated with hyaline membrane disease in full-term newborns.

1- Identify the factors predisposing to this pathology in order to establish a care and prevention strategy.

We conducted a retrospective descriptive study in the neonatology and neonatal intensive care unit of the main military training hospital in Tunis. We collated 34 newborns with MMH admitted to our department over a 3-year period from 1 January 2014 to 31 December 2016. Newborns admitted from the delivery room of the gynaecology-obstetrics department of the HMPIT are called "In born". Out born" newborns are transferred to our department from another public or private health facility after prior telephone agreement. During the study period, we included all newborns whose gestational age was greater than or equal to 37 completed weeks of amenorrhoea, established by theoretical calculation of the term from the first day of the last menstrual period, or at Based on early ultrasound data taken before 12 weeks' amenorrhoea each time this examination has been carried out.Clinical evaluation of term at birth using morphological criteria was used as a secondary criterion for assessing term. Our study did not include all newborns whose gestational age was strictly less than 37 weeks of amenorrhoea by theoretical calculation of the term or by estimation based on morphological criteria, and newborns with malformations diagnosed ante- or post-natally.We adopted the diagnosis of MMH in newborns presenting with early-onset respiratory distress, with signs of retraction present at birth or from the first hour of life, with progressively worsening oxygen dependence associated or not with cyanosis. Blood cultures from the first 72 hours were negative.The radiological criteria used to make the diagnosis were the combination of at least two of the following signs: Poor lung expansion, a diffuse and symmetrical alveolar syndrome with a homogeneous decrease in the transparency of the lung parenchyma, with or without an air bronchogram. Clinical data were collected by consulting the medical records of newborns admitted to our department during the study period, and we filled in a form containing data relating to the mother, the course of the pregnancy and delivery, and clinical data relating to the newborn from birth to the end of care in our department (Appendix 1).

Epidemiological study :

- During the study period, the neonatology and neonatal intensive care unit of the HMPIT recorded 272 admissions of full-term neonates presenting with neonatal respiratory distress. MMH was diagnosed in 34 of these cases, representing a frequency of 12.5%.

- The mean age of the mothers was 33.18±4.6 years, ranging from 27 and 43. 61.7% were aged between 27 and 34.

- The mean parity was 2.56±1.02 with extremes between 1 and 5. 76.4%

were poor.

- The majority of women had no previous medical history.
- All the pregnancies were spontaneous, monochorionic and well monitored.
- Gestational diabetes was detected in all women. It was present in 20.5% of cases. Insulin-dependent diabetes prior to pregnancy was present in 5.8% of women.

- Antenatal corticosteroid therapy was administered to three women, only one of whom received two full courses and two of whom received a single course.

- Amniotic fluid was clear in 32 women. One woman had stained fluid and one woman had meconium fluid.

- The majority of newborns included in our study were "out born" with a frequency of 58.9%. The sex ratio was 1.6.

- The mean gestational age at birth was 38.12±0.96 SA with a range of between 37 and 41 SA.
- Cold caesarean section was scheduled in 82% of women. Emergency caesarean section was indicated in 8.8% of women for the following reasons: spontaneous onset of labour in a scarred uterus, chorioamniotitis and severe pre-eclampsia.

Clinical study :

- All neonates had a good adaptation to extra-uterine life. The mean Apgar at 5 minutes was 9.51±0.75 with extremes between 7 and 10.

- The mean birth weight was 3306±520g with extremes between 2170 and 4600g.

- The average age of newborns on admission was 12.05±14.25 hours. The "out born" were 19.15±14.43 hours old. The average age of the inborns was 1.57±1.09 hours.

- Respiratory distress was immediate in all neonates.

- Cyanosis was present in 35.2% of newborns.

- The mean Silvermann score on admission was 4.46±1.57 with a range of between 2 and 6.

- The average time taken to obtain chest X-rays was 10.85±12.43 hours, with extremes of between 1 and 43 hours.

- Chest X-rays showed an alveolar syndrome in 91.1% of cases. EGIT was present in 17.6% of cases.

- The average time taken to perform blood gas measurements was 14.59±15.08 hours, with extremes of between 0.5 and 50 hours.

- All neonates received mechanical ventilation. The mean age was of 16.88±14.46 hours.

- All neonates were treated with exogenous surfactant by instillation through the tracheal intubation tube. The mean age was 21.85±17.39 hours.

- High-frequency oscillatory ventilation was indicated for refractory hypoxaemia in 26.5% of cases. The mean age was 49.77±18.84 hours. The mean duration of HFO ventilation was 47.66±44.37 hours.

- EGIT occurred in 32.3% of newborns. Pneumothorax occurred in 16% of cases. Pneumomediastinum was noted in 16.3% of cases.

- Pulmonary arterial hypertension was found in 58% of cases. The use of nitric oxide was indicated in all cases of PAH at a mean age of 52.67±23.76 hours.

- The average length of hospital stay was 10.17±7.6 days.

- In 64% of newborns, discharge was without sequelae.

- Convulsions and hypotonia were noted in 23.5% of cases.

- Four newborns died of pulmonary hypertension in 3 cases and DIC in one case, related to a healthcare-associated infection.

Few studies have investigated MMH in the term newborn. This may be explained by the difficulty of eliminating other pathologies with the same clinico-radiological characteristics as MMH. Infectious alveolitis or transient respiratory distress are more easily evoked.

The limitations of our study were the retrospective nature of the study, with a lack of precision in some of the medical record data, the heterogeneity of the study population and the inclusion of "out born" neonates, which led to a selection bias, and the unavailability of in utero fetal lung maturation tests.

In our study, we found a male predominance, with a high rate of scheduled cold caesarean sections outside labour. This finding is consistent with the literature. Indeed, these two conditions are the most incriminated in the genesis of MMH in term newborns.Little is known about the role played by the degree of lung maturation in triggering labour and uterine contractions in parturients. Some authors have shown that certain foetuses are not mature at 37-38 weeks' gestation. Thus, failure to expose these foetuses to the stress of childbirth may be the cause of a functional surfactant deficiency.

Delays in the diagnosis and management of this condition, due to a lack of awareness of the entity, are a source of complications that can be serious, with severe sequelae. In fact, the assessment of respiratory distress using the Silvermann score is the main source of this delay. The score is low because of the rigid musculature of the term newborn.Intensive care management of neonates presenting with respiratory distress must always take into consideration the possibility of diagnosing MMH in full-term neonates. Management is based on oxygen therapy using mechanical ventilation with positive pressure, combined with replacement of surfactant deficiency by intra-tracheal instillation of exogenous surfactant. At the end of our study and in view of the data in the literature, we recommend:

- T o favour vaginal delivery whenever the conditions are right. maternal
obstetrics allow it.
- Reduce as far as possible the frequency of cold caesarean births outside
labour and delay fetal extraction beyond 39 weeks' gestation whenever
possible.

- To promote research in Tunisia to ensure the degree of lung maturation by
biochemical tests whenever extraction is envisaged before 39-40 SA.

- To limit or avoid, through coordinated obstetric and paediatric
management, the multiple factors likely to aggravate the functional
surfactant deficit at birth (acute foetal distress, inhalation, hypothermia,
maternal-foetal infection, cardiocirculatory insufficiency).

- To ensure optimal management in the intensive care unit with early
administration of exogenous surfactant whenever the diagnosis of MMH is
suspected in a newborn at term.

REFERENCES

[1]- Dehan M, Francoual J. Etiology of neonatal respiratory distress syndrome and the assessment of lung maturity. Ann Arbor, Boston: CRC Press Inc. 1991;4:333-58.

[2] Peschechera R, Andrisani MC, Reale F, Ciavarella C, Campioni P, Rays V. Diagnostic imaging of hyaline membrane disease. 2004;29(2):175-8.

[3]- Anadkat JS, Kuzniewicz MW, Chaudhari BP, Cole FS, Hamvas A. Increased risk for respiratory distress among white, male, late preterm and term infants. J perinatol. 2012;32(10):780-5.

[4]- Jonguitud AA. Elective caesarean section: impact of evolution neonatal respiration. Gynecol Obstet Mex. 2011;79(4):206-13.

[5]- Flamein F, Borie R, Epaud R. Hereditary surfactant pathologies: from birth to retirement. La lettre du pneumologue. 2013;2:62-7.

[6]- Zupan V, Lacaze-Masmonteil T. Le surfactant pulmonaire : de la physiopathologie à la thérapeutique. Sciences. 1993;9:277-87.

[7]- Magny JF, Rigourd V, Kieffer F, Voyer M. Corticothérapie périnatale : modalités, efficacité, conséquences. Jour gyn obst biol reprod. 2001;30:36-46.

[8]- Becquet O, El Khabbaz F, Alberti C, Mohamed D, Blachier A, Biran V, et al. Insulin-treated gestational diabetes and risk of severe respiratory distress in neonates older than 34 weeks of amenorrhea. Arch ped. 2016;23(3):261-7.

[9]- Lloreda-García JM, Sevilla-Denia S, Rodríguez-Sánchez A, Muñoz-Martínez P, Díaz-Ruiz M. Perinatal outcome of macrosomic infants born to diabetic versus non-diabetic mothers. Endocrinol Nutr. 2016;63(8):409-13.

[10]- Blondel B, Kermarrec M. Enquête nationale périnatale 2010 [On line]. Unité de Recherches Epidémiologiques en Santé Périnatale et la Santé des Femmes et des Enfants, INSERM- U.953, Paris. Available at URL: http://gynerisq.fr/wp- content/uploads/2013/12/2010-Enquete-Nationale-Périnatale.pdf.

[11]- Davies GA, Maxwell C, McLeod L, Gagnon R, Basso M, Bos H, et al. Obesity in pregnancy. J Obstet Gynaecol Can. 2010;32(2):165-73.

[12]- Dónaldsson SF, Dagbjartsson A, Bergsteinsson H, Hardardóttir H, Haraldsson A, Thórkelsson T . Respiratory dysfunction in infants born by elective cesarean section without labor. Laeknabladid. 2007;93(10):675-9.

[13]- Ramachandrappa A, Lucky Jain MBA. Elective Cesarean Section: It's Impact on Neonatal Respiratory Outcome. Clin Perinatol. 2008;35(2):373-93.

[14]- Alderdice F, McCall E, Bailie C, Craig S, Dornan J, McMillen R, et al. Admission to neonatal intensive care with respiratory morbidity following term elective caesarean section. Ir Med J. 2005;98:170-4.

[15]- Donaldsson SF, Dagbjartsson A, Bergsteinsson H, Hardardóttir H, Haraldsson A, Thórkelsson T. Respiratory dysfunction in infants born by elective cesarean section without labor. Laeknabladid. 2007;93(10):675-9.

[16]- Gerten KA, Coonrod DV, Bay RC, Chambliss LR. Cesarean delivery and respiratory distress syndrome: does labor make a difference? Am J Obstet Gynecol. 2005;193(3):1061-4.

[17]- Hansen AK, Wisborg K, Uldbjerg N, Henriksen TB. Risk of respiratory morbidity in term infants delivered by elective caesarean section: cohort study. BMJ. 2008;336(7635):85-7.

[18]- Kolas T, Saugstad OD, Daltveit AK, Nilsen ST, Øian P. Planned cesarean versus planned vaginal delivery at term: comparison of newborn

infant outcomes. Am J Obstet Gynecol. 2006;195(6):1538-43.

[19]- Richardson BS, Czikk MJ, daSilva O, Natale R. The impact of labor at term on measures of neonatal outcome. Am J Obstet Gynecol. 2005;192(1):219-26.

[20]- Jain L, Eaton DC. Physiology of fetal lung fluid clearance and the effect of labor. Semin Perinatol. 2006;30(1):34-43.

[21]- Alfirevic Z, Milan SJ, Livio S. Caesarean section versus vaginal delivery for preterm birth in singletons. Cochrane Database Syst Rev. 2013;(9):CD000078.

[22]- Wankaew N, Jirapradittha J, Kiatchoosakun P. Neonatal morbidity and mortality for repeated cesarean section vs normal vaginal delivery to uncomplicated term pregnancies at Srinagarind Hospital. J Med Assoc Thai. 2013;96(6):654-60.

[23]- Chiossi G, Lai Y, Landon MB, Spong CY, Rouse DJ, Varner MW, et al. Timing of delivery and adverse outcomes in term singleton repeat cesarean deliveries. Obstet Gynecol. 2013;121(3):561-9.

[24]- Gluck L, Kulovich MV, Borer RC, Brenner PH, Anderson GG, Spellacy WN. Diagnosis of the respiratory distress syndrome by amniocentesis. Am J Obstet Gynecol. 1971;109:440-5.

[25]- Shinitzky M, Goldfisher A, Bruck A, Goldman B, Stern E, Barkai G, et al. A new method for assessment of fetal lung maturity. Br J Obstet Gynecol. 1976;83:838-44.

[26]- Ayachi A, Rigourd V, Kieffer F, Dommergues MA, Voyer M, Magny JF. Hyaline membrane disease in term newborns. Arch ped. 2005;12:156-9.

[27]- Ertuğrul S, Gün I, Müngen E, Muhçu M, Kılıç S, Atay V. Evaluation

of neonatal outcomes in elective repeat cesarean delivery at term according to weeks of gestation. J Obstet Gynecol Res. 2013;39(1):105-12.

[28]- Wax JR, Herson V, Carignan E, Mather J, Ingardia JC. Contribution of elective delivery to severe respiratory distress at term. Amer J Perinatol. 2002;19(2):81-6.

[29]- Doan E, Gibbons K, Tudehope D. The timing of elective caesarean deliveries and early neonatal outcomes in singleton infants born 37-41 weeks' gestation. ANZJOG. 2014;54(6):602-5.

[30]- Rodriguez A, Viscardi RM, Torday JS. Fetal androgen exposure inhibits fetal rat lung fibroblast lipid uptake and release. Exp Lung Res. 2001;27(1):13-24.

[31]- Nielsen HC, Zinman HM, Torday JS. Dihydrotestosterone inhibits fetal rabbit pulmonary surfactant production. J Clin Invest. 1982;69(3):611-6.

[32]- Martin JA. Births: final data for 2004. Natl Vital Stat Rep. 2006;55(1):110-1. [33] Pérez Molina JJ, Blancas Jacobo O, Ramírez Valdivia JM. Hyaline membrane
disease: mortality and maternal and neonatal risk factors. Ginecol Obstet Mex. 2006;74(7):354-9.

[34]- Stein HM, Martinez A, Blount L, Oyama K, Padbury JF. The effects of corticosteroids and thyrotropin-releasing hormone on newborn adaptation and sympathoadrenal in preterm sheep. Am J Obstet Gynecol. 1994,171:17-24.

[35]- Gouyon C, Ribakovsky C, Ferdynus C, Quantin P, Sagot B, Burgundy G. Severe respiratory disorders in term neonates. Paediatr perinat epidemiol. 2008;22(1):22-30.

[36]- Liu J, Shi Y, Dong JY, Zheng T, Li JY, Lu L, et al. Clinical characteristics, diagnosis and management of respiratory distress syndrome in full-term neonates. Chin Med J. 2010;123(19):2640-4.

[37]- Bouziri A, Ben Slima S, Hamdi A, Menif K, Belhadj S, Khaldi A, et al. Acute respiratory distress syndrome in infants at term and near term about 23 cases. Tunis Med. 2007;85: 874-9.

[37]- DeMello DE, Heyman S, Phelps DS. Ultrastructure of lung in surfactant protein B deficiency. Am J Respir Cell Mol Biol. 1994;11:230-9.

[39]- Nogee LM, Garnier G, Dietz HC. Mutation in the surfactant protein B gene responsible for fatal neonatal resiratory disease in multiple kindreds. J Clin Invest. 1994;93(4):1860-3.

[40]- Nogee LM, Dunbar AE, 3rd, Wert SE, Askin F, Hamvas A, Whitsett JA. A mutation in the surfactant protein C gene associated with familial interstitial lung disease. N Engl J Med. 2001;344(8):573-9.

[41]- Bridges JP, Xu Y, Na CL. Adaptation and increased susceptibility to infection associated with constitutive expression of misfolded SP-C. J Cell Biol. 2006;172:395-407.

[42]- Bullard JE, Nogee LM. Heterozygosity for ABCA3 mutations modifies the severity of lung disease associated with a surfactant protein C gene (SFTPC) mutation. Pediatr Res. 2007;62(2):176-9.

[43] - Escande B, Kuhn P, Rivera S, Messer J. Secondary surfactant deficiency. EMC-Médecine. 2005; 2(5):554-69.

[44]- Bhuta T, Kent-Biggs J, Jeffery HE. Prediction of surfactant dysfunction in term infants by the click test. Pediatr Pulmonol. 1997;23(4):287-91.

[45]- NooriShadkam M, Lookzadeh MH, Taghizadeh M, Golzar A, NooriShadkam Z. Diagnostic value of gastric shake test for hyaline membrane disease in preterm infant. Iran J Reprod Med. 2014;12(7):487-91.

[46]- Post M. Maternal administration of dexamethasone stimulates cholinephosphate cytidyltransferase in fetal type II cells. Biochem J. 1987;241:291-6.

[47]- Morales WJ, Diebel ND, Lazar AJ, Zadrozny D. The effect of antenatal dexamethasone on the prevention of respiratory distress syndrome. Am J Obstet Gynecol. 1986;154:591-5.

[48]- Gamsu HR, Mullinger BM, Donnai P, Dash CH. Antenatal administration of betamethasone to prevent respiratory distress syndrome in preterm infants: report of a UK multicentre trial. Br J Obstet Gynecol. 1989;96:401-10.

[49]- Collaborative group on antenatal steroid therapy. Effect of antenatal dexamethasone administration on the prevention of respiratory distress syndrome. Am J Obstet Gynecol. 1981;141:276-87.

[50]- Bourbon JR, Fraslon C. Developmental aspects of the alveolar epithelium and the pulmonary surfactant system in pulmonary surfactant: biochemical, functional, regulatory and clinical concepts. CRC Press. 1991:257-324.

[51]- Nada AM, Shafeek MM, El Maraghy MA, Nageeb AH, Salah El Din AS, Awad MH. Antenatal corticosteroid administration before elective caesarean section at term to prevent neonatal respiratory morbidity: a randomized controlled trial. Eur J Obstet Gynecol Reprod Biol. 2016;199:88-91.

[52]- Pctour Gazitúa F, Pérez Velásquez J. Do antenatal corticosteroids in

term elective cesarean sections reduce neonatal respiratory morbidity? Medwave. 2015;15(9):62-80.

[53]- Ahmed MR, Sayed Ahmed WA, Mohammed TY. Antenatal steroids at 37 weeks, does it reduce neonatal respiratory morbidity? A randomized trial. J Matern Fetal Neonatal Med. 2015;28(12):1486-90.

[54]- Stutchfield PR, Zbaeda M, Furneaux L, Satelle J, Banfield P, Bickerton NJ, et al. Antenatal steroid therapy for elective caesarean section at birth. Arch Dis Child. 2004;89(1):4-7.

[55]- Saccone G, Berghella V. Antenatal corticosteroids for maturity of term or near term fetuses: systematic review and meta-analysis of randomized controlled trials. BMJ. 2016;12:355-9.

[56]- Whitsett JA. Respiratory Distress Syndrome-Hyaline Membrane. Sciences. 2014;3:12-7.

[57]- Fujiwara T, Chida S, Watabe Y, Mreta H, Morita T, Abc T. Artificial surfactant therapy in hyaline membrane disease. Lancet. 1980;1:55-9.

[58]- Goraya JS, Nada R, Ray M. Hyaline membrane disease in a term neonate.Indian J Pediatr. 2001;68(8):771-3.

[59]- Merritt TA, Hallman M, Berry C, Pohjavuori M, Edwards DK, Jaaskelainen J, et al. Randomized, placebo-controlled trial of human surfactant given at birth versus reseue administration in very low birth weight infants with lung immaturity. J Pediatr. 1991;118:581-94.

[60]- The Osiris collaborative group. Early versus delayed neonatal administration of a synthetic surfactant: the judgement of Osiris. Lancet. 1992;340:1363-9.

[61]- Bahadue FL, Soll R. Early versus delayed selective surfactant treatment for neonatal respiratory distress syndrome. Cochrane Database

Syst Rev. 2012;11:65-9.

[62]- Soll R, Ozek E. Multiple versus single doses of exogenous surfactant for the prevention or treatment of neonatal respiratory distress syndrome. Cochrane Database of Systematic Reviews. 2009:1;CD000141.

[63]- Judith U, Hibbard M, Wilkins I, Sun L, Kimberly G, Matthew H, et al. Respiratory morbidity in late preterm births. JAMA. 2010;28(4):419-425.

[64]- European Exosurf Study Group. Early or selective surfactant (Colfosceril Palmitate, Exosurf) for intubated babies at 26 to 29 weeks gestation: a European double-blind trial with sequential analysis. Online Journal of Current Clinical Trials. 1992;28:123-34.

[65]- Hentschel R, Dittrich F, Hilgendorff A, Wauer R, Westmeier M, Gortner L. Neurodevelopmental outcome and pulmonary morbidity two years after early versus late surfactant treatment: does it really differ? Acta Pediatric. 2009;98(4):654-9.

[66]- Advances in the diagnosis and management of persistent pulmonary hypertension of the newborn. Pediatr Clin North Am. 2009;56:579-600.

[67]- Abdel Mohsen AK, and Amin AS. Risk Factors and Outcomes of Persistent Pulmonary Hypertension of the Newborn in Neonatal Intensive Care Unit of Al- Minya University Hospital in Egypt. J Clin Neonatol. 2013;2(2):78-82.

[68]- Sirageldin MK, Selma MA , Abdelhaleem N. Neonatal respiratory distress in Omdurman Maternity Hospital, Sudan. J Paediatr. 2014;14(1):65-70.

[69]- Kumar A, Bhat Bv. Respiratory distress in newborn. Indian J Matern child Health. 1996;7:8-10.

[70]- Qian LL, Liu CQ, Guo YX, Jiang YJ. Current status of neonatal acute respiratory disorders. Chin Med J. 2010;123:2769-75.

[71]- Rubaltelli FF, Dani C, Reali MF, Bertini G, Wiechmann L, Tangucci M, Spagnolo A. Acute neonatal respiratory distress in Italy. Acta Paediatr. 1998;87:1261-8.

APPENDICES

Appendix 1: Study sheet

Identification :

Name:

DM

Sex : M / F inborn : yes / No

Mother:

Age

Parity

MEDICAL HISTORY

Pregnancy:

Spontaneous: yes / nomonofetal: yes / no

$\geq$ 3 echoes. : yes /no Diabetes:(0: no diabetes, 1: GDM, 2: type 1, 3: type 2)

If diabetes, Balanced: ...... (0: Not balanced,1: diet, 2: insulin)

Toxemia: yes / no anaemia : yes / no Dexa :(0, 1,2,3,4)

Time to delivery (H):

Giving birth :

GA: (1d=0.14)Presentation: C / S / other. RPM: yes / no

Liquid :C / T / M/ SFunicular anomaly:(0: None, 1: HRP 2: PP, 3: other)

RCF(0 : Not done, 1 : normal, 2 : dip I, 3 : dip II, 3 : a reactive, 4 :

tachycardiaFetal)

Mat. fever($\geq$ 38.5 /24h before acc.): yes / noSyndrome infl. Mat (20/15000):

yes / no

Channel:(0: VBNI, 1: VBI, 2: CSF, 3: CSW)

Indication (if cs)

Anaesthesia :P / G

Birth :

PN g trophicity (0 : Eutrophic, 1 : hyper, 2 : IUGR) Apgar 5' RSDN :(0 :
None, 1 : VPP, 2 : VPP+MCE, 3 : SDN intubation)

DRNN :

Immediate: yes / no

Age PEC (h)

SS

FR :

Sat O2

HD: (0: good, 1: bad)

Neuro:(0 : Good, 1 : Bad) S.Associés

Rx time % birth (h): .

Rx signs (0 : normal, 1 : scissuritis, 2 path. Alv, 3 : EGIT)

Delays GDS :

PH :

PCO2

Oxygen therapy :

	Age (H)	Indication	Duration (H)
Hood			
CPAP			
NIV			
VACI			
OHF			

Surfactant:yes / noAge (surf.) In H

Complications :

Ep.G.I.Th :yes / nodelay (EGIT)h:

Mode V :

Tr. Ventilation : yes / no

PAH: yes / no HCAI (ATB x5d): yes / no

HD distress (VA drugs): yes / no

Evolution :

Length of stay (days)

Outcome(0: discharge without sequelae,1: discharge with sequelae, 2: death)

sequelae

Cause death

Appendix 2: Apgar score

Quotation	Heartbeats	Breathing	Colour	Muscle tone	Reactivity to stimulation
0	Absent	Absent	Blue or pale	None	None
1	< 100/min	A few spontaneous movements	Cyanosis of the extremities	Hypotonia	Grimaces
2	>100/min	Normal	Rose	Normal tone	Cris

Appendix 3: Silvermann score

Criteria	0	1	2
Nose flapping	Absent	Moderate	Intense
Drawing	Absent	Intercostal	Intercostal and suprasternal
Expiratory whine	Absent	With a stethoscope	By ear
Xiphoid funnel	Absent	Moderate	Intense
Thoraco-abdominal swing	Synchronous breathing	Motionless thorax	Paradoxical breathing

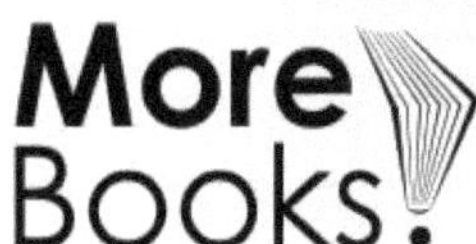

yes I want morebooks!

Buy your books fast and straightforward online - at one of world's fastest growing online book stores! Environmentally sound due to Print-on-Demand technologies.

Buy your books online at
www.morebooks.shop

Kaufen Sie Ihre Bücher schnell und unkompliziert online – auf einer der am schnellsten wachsenden Buchhandelsplattformen weltweit! Dank Print-On-Demand umwelt- und ressourcenschonend produziert.

Bücher schneller online kaufen
www.morebooks.shop

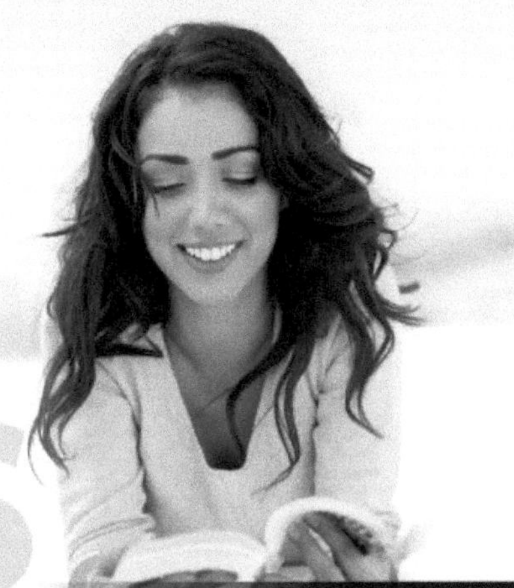

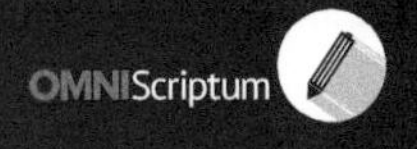

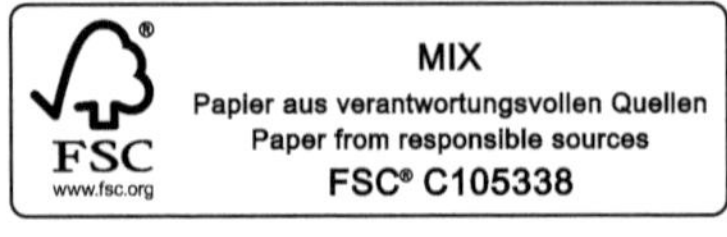

Printed by Books on Demand GmbH, Norderstedt / Germany